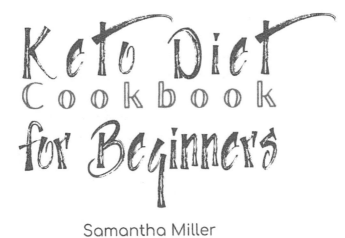

Keto Diet Cookbook for Beginners

Samantha Miller

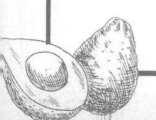
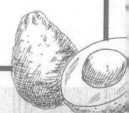

Table of Contents

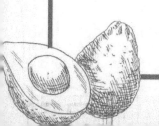
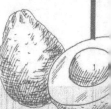

Introduction

The Ketogenic diet comprises the intake of high fat and low carbs. Drastically reducing the number of carbohydrates, ingesting, and replacing them with fat will put your body in ketosis. Ketosis is a metabolic state in which your body relies on fat for fuel instead of glucose in your blood. Macros or macronutrients are molecules our body uses to make energy. These comprise fat, protein, and carbs. Carbohydrates have 4 calories for every gram; fats, having 9 calories per gram. Lastly, protein comes in with 4 calories for every gram.

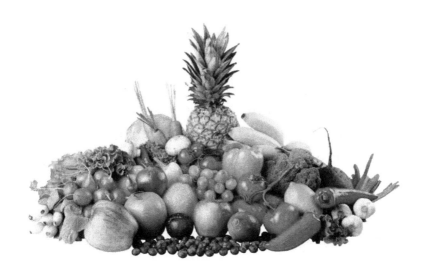

Naturally, counting calories and ingesting less of them will help you lose weight, but if not, be careful as you might not eat the right calories and may end up losing muscle mass. Counting macros instead can counter this. 100 calories of avocado (fat) are better than 100 calories of a doughnut (carb). With the Keto diet, it's important to be aware of your carbs-to-protein and fat ratio. Normally, to maintain ketosis, most people aim for 50 grams or fewer carbs a day.

When calculating macros, you just add up the grams of fat, carbs, and protein you ate that day. Let's say you had 10 saltine crackers, and a serving size is 5 crackers. You would then multiply the numbers on the label by 28g of fat, 20g of carbs, and 2g of protein. Document this process, and you can visually see where your number runs high in carbs.

There are several ways you can document your process, and you're encouraged to try all that work for you. You really will have to be diligent in this diet to ensure you're eating the proper proportion of macronutrients, and it may become endlessly helpful for you to keep track of your process—not to mention your day-to-day consumption.

You might consider just keeping tabs on your progress with a series of notes on your phone, but you may have a little more time to devote some careful attention to this procedure. In that case, you might try journaling about your intake, your process, and its outcomes. You may also feel drawn to using an app that could help you keep track of these same things. Finally, you could try using a dry erase board to keep tabs on your meal plan or menu for the week. More creative readers will extrapolate far more options beyond just these few provided.

No matter what you do, you're encouraged—at least for the first few weeks of your diet—to be conscientious of your food labels and keep track of what you're eating in a journal or an app. It's also good to have a scale for your household and a travel scale for the on-the-go. It's such that not all keto-friendly products have nutrition labels on them. It might be up to you to determine how much of what you're eating.

The keto diet is a very healthy and natural way to lose weight, but as with most new health regimens, there can be a rather lengthy period of change for some people—for some bodies, I should say. Truly, few will experience what we call the Keto-Flu during the beginning of the diet, and it typically lasts about a week, so don't be too concerned if you relate to these symptoms.

It occurs because the body is in a state similar to a shock from a drastic reduction to your regular carbohydrate intake. We have termed this syndrome of symptoms the Keto-Flu because the symptoms are like standard influenza. For instance, some of the symptoms include nausea, headache, and weakness. If you feel any of these symptoms, you must be very careful to watch out for sugar cravings. This craving, on top of everything else, may make you feel miserable, and it could even possibly make you want to quit. However, there are ways to reduce these rather frustrating symptoms.

First, drink plenty of water, during your keto diet. You will lose water weight, which is wonderful, except it increases your risk for dehydration. Keep drinking water to prevent muscle cramps and fatigue, which can be because of dehydration. Don't worry because you'll keep losing that water weight, so water taken in won't set you back at all.

Second, don't take part in any strenuous activity because your body needs to adjust to a fresh fuel source. You'll want to take time for yourself and relax, but if you want to exercise, do yoga or light walking more so than anything strenuous.

Third, make sure you are consuming enough fat. With a low-carb diet, your body will crave bread and sweets. Making sure you eat enough fat will help suppress the need for sweets that might take over your mind. These healthy fats will keep you sated, distracted, and satisfied, but if you struggle, you can also try to reduce carb intake slowly instead of cutting everything out all at once.

Fourth and last, you can become tired and irritable when adjusting to the keto diet. Adjusting one's diet is already enough to stress anyone out, but you will cut out large (formerly standard) parts of your diet. Be patient with yourself, and be sure to incorporate adequate time for sleep. Not enough sleep increases stress levels on top of everything else new you'll be sifting through, so ensure you get adequate amounts of sleep—particularly during your transition into this diet.

Achieving ketosis is not exactly easy, but if you follow the diet correctly and stay diligent, your body should shift into ketosis within two to six weeks. This amount of time is usually the adaptation phase.

We recommend no definite amount of time to do the Keto diet. Navigating around carbs is hard, especially around gatherings and holidays. But as long as you are mindful and know how to balance meals, you can slowly introduce carbs back into your diet.

There are many benefits to following the Keto diet. Naturally, it aids greatly in how fast you can lose weight. The high protein in the diet keeps you full longer. It reduces acne. Countless studies show that diet can affect your skin health, so refining your diet and not taking in carbs and sugars increases the health of your skin.

It's good for your heart because it reduces the risk of heart disease. On the keto diet, your cholesterol is affected positively, too, and it is called LDL decreases. That's essentially bad cholesterol. HDL increases, on the other hand, is good cholesterol. Additionally, it can improve the health of women with PCOS through weight loss and improving hormone balancing.

Starting the Keto diet and living the Keto lifestyle doesn't have to be hard. There are a plethora of meals you can prepare for your week. Meals in this book are affordable and easy to make, saving you time and money all in four steps.

Have a shopping list ready based on what you want to cook for that week. Here are some foods you can buy:

• Meats—almost all meat is good for a keto diet, especially if it's high in fat. Watch your sausage and portions of bacon because these can have added carbs and sugars for flavor. Go for uncured meats. Beef, chuck roast, poultry, pork, venison brats, hot dogs, etc.

- Veggies & fruits—many will argue that a lot of vegetables are off the table because of carb content. As such, you have to look for veggies with lower carbs and high fiber content. Broccoli, cauliflower, bell pepper, cucumbers, spaghetti squash, avocados, and berries are good choices; just be sure to watch your sugar and carb intake.

- Dairy—we recommend Milk for the keto diet; however, full-fat cheeses and other dairy products are also ok. Just always look at your nutrition labels because the nutrition content varies in almost every brand. Anything from Greek yogurt to butter, cheese (hard varieties), heavy whipping cream, cream cheese, sour cream, and even eggs is acceptable.

- Oils & fats—Keto is often considered as a high-fat diet, but use your fats wisely, and that includes the oils used for cooking. Avoid vegetable and canola oil. Seek for oils like coconut, sesame, olive, and avocado instead.

- Flour & grains—You'll see this in a lot of these recipes that call for almond flour, flax meal, chia seeds, etc. We can find most of these at your local grocery stores. In some stores, you can just buy the amount you need by the pound.

1. Make Your Way to the Store

Shopping for a diet plan can be overwhelming, and hard to get the best bang for your buck. For your vegetables and fruits, check out any local market or farm stand. Most of those products will be fresh and unprocessed. Also, visit your local ethnic and Hispanic markets, for they often carry products you can't find at your farmers' market or store. Buy in bulk so you can keep produce that isn't in season, and freeze it until you're ready to use it. For your meats, many grocery stores will put out meats and poultry they need to sell quickly out at a discount. We usually do this on weekends in the early morning, but you may check with your grocery stores. You can also visit butcher shops to buy meat in bulk to get a good price.

Once you have your shopping and your ingredients prepared, you can start with your prep.

If you want to change it up in the middle of the week, the suggested days to meal-prep are Sundays and Wednesdays. Make sure your prep area is clean. Layout enough ingredients according to the number of days you want to have the meal ready for. Have your containers ready and any kitchen utensils, pots, or pans you'll use out. Start by cooking any meat, fish, and/or poultry you have, as this can take the longest time.

As you prepare meals, begin adding, chopping, and assembling any other ingredient you have into your containers. Add your meat after and store. It's wise to have a designated spot in your refrigerator for your prepped meals.

There are several utensils and appliances you will read about in the recipes, such are graters, spiralizers, and blenders. You can find these items at your local Wal-Mart or grocery for relatively low prices. Also, you can find hand and box grates at most dollar stores. You can use a hand mixer instead of a blender most of the time. However, you might need it in some dishes.

There are also a lot of subsites for ingredients, such as the xanthan gum, which is a sub for cornstarch and is a thickening agent, and erythritol, which is a sugar sub. These can be difficult to find in stores but are easy to find online and easy on the wallet.

Almost all the recipes in this book are perfect for meal prep. Portion all pieces of your meals and keep them in airtight containers. Reheating is easy; just pop them in the microwave for a minute or two. If there are aspects of the meal that need to be under heat by itself, just cover them with a damp paper towel.

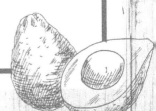

Breakfast Recipes

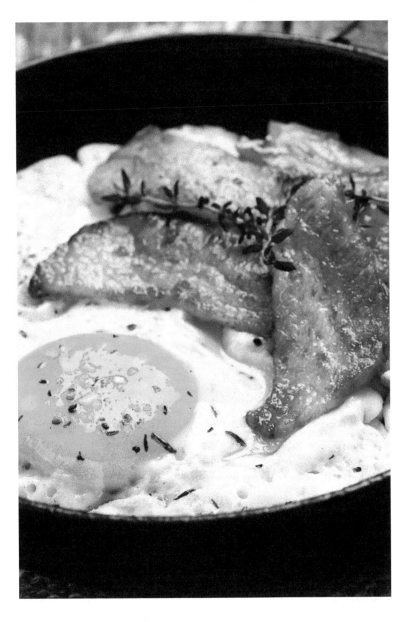

Prep time:– 10 min; Servings: - 5

INGREDIENTS:

1 zucchini

½ avocado

20 basil leaves

1 Tbsp olive oil

3 brown mushrooms

1 garlic clove

1 tsp lemon juice

¼ tsp salt

DIRECTIONS:

Spiralize zucchini.

Slice the mushrooms in half.

Place avocado, basil, ½ Tbsp olive oil, garlic, lemon juice and salt in a stick blender cup. Blend for about a minute.

In a frying pan, add ½ Tbsp olive oil and cook until tender. Add the zucchini noodles and cook until they get warm for just a minute or so.

NUTRITION: 383 Cal, 35.34g fat, 18g carbs, 5.46g protein

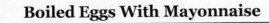

2   Boiled Eggs With Mayonnaise

Prep time:- 10 min; Servings: - 4

INGREDIENTS:

8 eggs

8 Tbsp mayonnaise

2 avocados (optional)

DIRECTIONS:

Boil water in a pot

Optional: use an egg piercer to make tiny holes in the shells which help eggs crack as they cook.

Carefully place the eggs in the pot.

For soft-boiled eggs, boil for 5-6 min, for medium-boiled eggs 6-8 min and for hard-boiled eggs 8-10 min

Serve with mayonnaise.

NUTRITION: Cal 316 , Protein 11g, Fat 29g, Net Carbs 1g

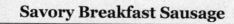

3 Savory Breakfast Sausage

Prep time:– 10min; Servings: – 4

INGREDIENTS:

¼ tsp cayenne pepper

1 tsp sage

220g ground chicken

220g ground pork

¼ tsp celery seed, nutmeg, garlic powder, onion powder and paprika

½ tsp salt, black pepper

DIRECTIONS:

Mix all the ingredients in a bowl and knead with your hands.

Make 6 hamburger patties and fry on both sides over medium heat.

NUTRITION: 185 Cal, 12.81g fat, 0.25g carbs, 16.17g protein

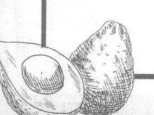
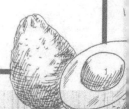

4   Avocado Eggs With Bacon Sails

Prep time:- 15 - 20 min; Servings: − 4

INGREDIENTS:

2 medium eggs, hard-boiled

½ avocado

1 Tbsp olive oil

2 medium slices of bacon

Salt and pepper to taste

DIRECTIONS:

Boil the eggs and let them cool

Take out the yolks and mix with the avocado, oil and salt and pepper.

Fry the bacon for 5 -7 min until crispy.

With a spoon, carefully add the mixture back into the egg and set the bacon sail.

NUTRITION: : Cal 157 , Fat 14g, Protein 6g, Net carbs 1g

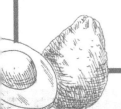

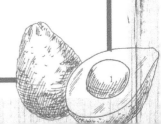

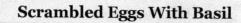

5   Scrambled Eggs With Basil

Prep time:5-7 min; Servings: – 1

INGREDIENTS:

2 Tbsp coconut cream or coconut milk

½ tsp salt

1 oz butter

2 oz shredded cheese (optional)

2 Tbsp fresh basil, chopped

2 eggs

DIRECTIONS:

Melt the butter over low heat.

In a small bowl, mix the egg whites, basil coconut cream/milk and salt.

Gently whisk the mixture, pour into the pan and scramble.

NUTRITION: Fat 42g, Protein13g, Net carbs 2g, Cal 427

Snack & Appetizer Recipes

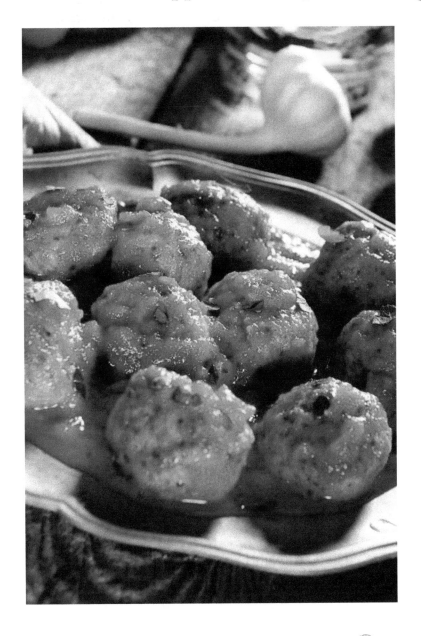

6   Dijon Beef Meatball and Cheese Kebabs

Prep time: 20 minutes | Cook time: 15 minutes |
Serves 4

INGREDIENTS:

1 tablespoon Dijon mustard
2 tablespoons minced scallions
1 pound ground beef
1½ teaspoons minced green garlic
½ teaspoon cumin
Salt and ground black pepper, to taste
12 cherry tomatoes
12 cubes Cheddar cheese

DIRECTIONS:

In a large-sized mixing dish, place the mustard,
ground beef, cumin, scallions, garlic, salt, and pepper;
mix with your hands or a spatula so that everything is
evenly coated.

Form into 12 meatballs and cook them in the
preheated Air Fryer for 15 minutes at 375°F (190°C).
Air-fry until they are cooked in the middle.

Thread cherry tomatoes, mini burgers and cheese on
cocktail sticks. Bon appétit!

NUTRITION: calories: 469 | fat: 30g | protein: 3g |
carbs: 4g | net carbs: 3g

7   Cheddar Prosciutto Pierogi

Prep time: 15 minutes | Cook time: 20 minutes | Makes 4 pierogi

INGREDIENTS:

1 cup chopped cauliflower

2 tablespoons diced onions

1 tablespoon unsalted butter, melted

Pinch of fine sea salt

½ cup shredded sharp Cheddar cheese (about 2 ounces)

8 slices prosciutto

Fresh oregano leaves, for garnish (optional)

DIRECTIONS:

Preheat the air fryer to 350°F (180°C). Lightly grease a 7-inch pie pan or a casserole dish that will fit in your air fryer.

Make the filling: Place the cauliflower and onion in the pan. Drizzle with the melted butter and sprinkle with the salt. Using your hands, mix everything together, making sure the cauliflower is coated in the butter.

Place the cauliflower mixture in the air fryer and cook for 10 minutes, until fork-tender, stirring halfway through.

Transfer the cauliflower mixture to a food processor or high-powered blender. Spray the air fryer basket with avocado oil and increase the air fryer temperature to 400°F (205°C).

Pulse the cauliflower mixture in the food processor until smooth. Stir in the cheese.

Assemble the pierogi: Lay 1 slice of prosciutto on a sheet of parchment paper with a short end toward you. Lay another slice of prosciutto on top of it at a right angle, forming a cross. Spoon about 2 heaping tablespoons of the filling into the center of the cross. Fold each arm of the prosciutto cross over the filling to form a square, making sure that the filling is well covered. Using your fingers, press down around the filling to even out the square shape. Repeat with the rest of the prosciutto and filling.

Spray the pierogi with avocado oil and place them in the air fryer basket. Cook for 10 minutes, or until crispy.

Garnish with oregano before serving, if desired. Store leftovers in an airtight container in the fridge for up to 4 days. Reheat in a preheated 400°F (205°C) air fryer for 3 minutes, or until heated through.

NUTRITION: calories: 150 | fat: 11g | protein: 11g | carbs: 2g | net carbs: 1g

8   Spinach Melts with Parsley Yogurt Dip

Prep time: 20 minutes | Cook time: 14 minutes |
Serves 4

INGREDIENTS:

Spinach Melts:

2 cups spinach, torn into pieces

1 ½ cups cauliflower

1 tablespoon sesame oil

½ cup scallions, chopped

2 garlic cloves, minced

½ cup almond flour

¼ cup coconut flour

1 teaspoon baking powder

½ teaspoon sea salt

½ teaspoon ground black pepper

¼ teaspoon dried dill

½ teaspoon dried basil

1 cup Cheddar cheese, shredded

Parsley Yogurt Dip:

½ cup Greek-Style yoghurt

2 tablespoons mayonnaise

2 tablespoons fresh parsley, chopped

1 tablespoon fresh lemon juice

½ teaspoon garlic, smashed

DIRECTIONS:

Place spinach in a mixing dish; pour in hot water. Drain and rinse well.

Add cauliflower to the steamer basket; steam until the cauliflower is tender about 5 minutes.

Mash the cauliflower; add the remaining ingredients for Spinach Melts and mix to combine well. Shape the mixture into patties and transfer them to the lightly greased cooking basket.

Bake at 330°F (166°C) for 14 minutes or until thoroughly heated.

Meanwhile, make your dipping sauce by whisking the remaining ingredients. Place in your refrigerator until ready to serve.

Serve the Spinach Melts with the chilled sauce on the side. Enjoy!

NUTRITION: calories: 301 | fat: 25g | protein: 11g | carbs: 9g | net carbs: 5g

9   Dill Pickle Spears with Ranch Dressing

Prep time: 40 minutes | Cook time: 10 minutes | Serves 4

INGREDIENTS:

4 dill pickle spears, halved lengthwise
¼ cup ranch dressing
½ cup blanched finely ground almond flour
½ cup grated Parmesan cheese
2 tablespoons dry ranch seasoning

DIRECTIONS:

Wrap spears in a kitchen towel 30 minutes to soak up excess pickle juice.

Pour ranch dressing into a medium bowl and add pickle spears. In a separate medium bowl, mix flour, Parmesan, and ranch seasoning.

Remove each spear from ranch dressing and shake off excess. Press gently into dry mixture to coat all sides. Place spears into ungreased air fryer basket. Adjust the temperature to 400°F (205°C) and set the timer for 10 minutes, turning spears three times during cooking. Serve warm.

NUTRITION: calories: 160 | fat: 11g | protein: 7g | carbs: 8g | net carbs: 6g

10 Parmesan Chicken Nuggets with Mayo

Prep time: 20 minutes | Cook time: 12 minutes | Serves 6

INGREDIENTS:

1 pound chicken breasts, slice into tenders

½ teaspoon cayenne pepper

Salt and black pepper, to taste

¼ cup almond meal

1 egg, whisked

½ cup Parmesan cheese, freshly grated

¼ cup mayo

¼ cup no-sugar-added barbecue sauce

DIRECTIONS:

Pat the chicken tenders dry with a kitchen towel. Season with the cayenne pepper, salt, and black pepper.

Dip the chicken tenders into the almond meal, followed by the egg. Press the chicken tenders into the Parmesan cheese, coating evenly.

Place the chicken tenders in the lightly greased Air Fryer basket. Cook at 360°F (182°C) for 9 to 12 minutes, turning them over to cook evenly.

In a mixing bowl, thoroughly combine the mayonnaise with the barbecue sauce. Serve the chicken nuggets with the sauce for dipping. Bon appétit!

NUTRITION: calories: 268 | fat: 18g | protein: 2g | carbs: 4g | net carbs: 3g

Poultry Recipes

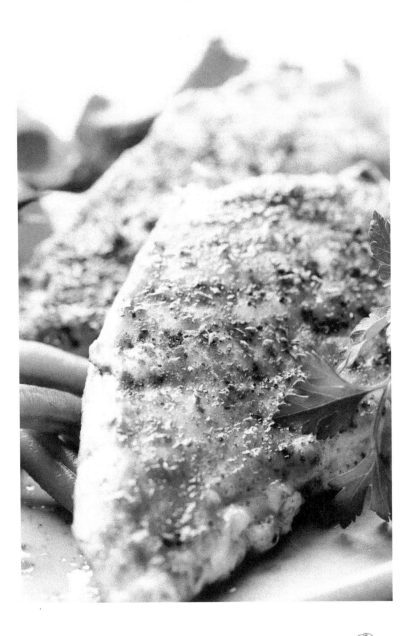

11   Italian-Style Chicken Meatballs with Parmesan

Ready in about 20 minutes | Servings 6

INGREDIENTS:

For the Meatballs:

1 ¼ pounds chicken, ground

1 tablespoon sage leaves, chopped

1 teaspoon shallot powder

1 teaspoon porcini powder

2 garlic cloves, finely minced

1/3 teaspoon dried basil

3/4 cup Parmesan cheese, grated

2 eggs, lightly beaten

Salt and ground black pepper, to your liking

1/2 teaspoon cayenne pepper

For the sauce:

2 tomatoes, pureed

1 cup chicken consommé

2 ½ tablespoons lard, room temperature

1 onion, peeled and finely chopped

DIRECTIONS:

In a mixing bowl, combine all ingredients the meatballs. Roll the mixture into bite-sized balls.

Melt 1 tablespoon of lard in a skillet over a moderately high heat. Sear the meatballs for about 3 minutes or until they are thoroughly cooked; reserve.

Melt the remaining lard and cook the onions until tender and translucent.

Add in pureed tomatoes and chicken consommé and continue to cook for 4 minutes longer.

Add in the reserved meatballs, turn the heat to simmer and continue to cook for 6 to 7 minutes.

Bon appétit!

NUTRITION: 252 Calories; 9.7g Fat; 5.3g Carbs; 34.2g Protein;

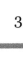
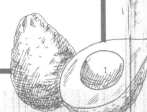

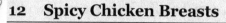

12   Spicy Chicken Breasts

Ready in about 30 minutes | Servings 6

INGREDIENTS:

1 ½ pounds chicken breasts

1 bell pepper, deveined and chopped

1 leek, chopped

1 tomato, pureed

2 tablespoons coriander

2 garlic cloves, minced

1 teaspoon cayenne pepper

1 teaspoon dry thyme

1/4 cup coconut aminos

Sea salt and ground black pepper, to taste

DIRECTIONS:

Rub each chicken breasts with the garlic, cayenne pepper, thyme, salt and black pepper.

Cook the chicken in a saucepan over medium-high heat.

Sear for about 5 minutes until golden brown on all sides.

Fold in the tomato puree and coconut aminos and bring it to a boil.

Add in the pepper, leek, and coriander.

Reduce the heat to simmer. Continue to cook, partially covered, for about 20 minutes.

Bon appétit!

NUTRITION: 239 Calories; 8.6g Fat; 5.5g Carbs; 34.3g Protein;

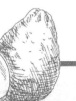

13 Roasted Chicken Kabobs with Celery Fries

Ready in about: 50 minutes | Serves: 4

INGREDIENTS:

1 lb chicken breasts, cubed
4 tbsp olive oil
1 cup chicken vegetable broth
1 head celery root, sliced
2 tbsp olive oil
Salt and black pepper to taste

DIRECTIONS:

Preheat oven to 400°F.

In a bowl, mix 2 tbsp of the olive oil, salt, and pepper. Add in the chicken and toss to coat. Cover with foil and place in the fridge.

Arrange the celery slices in a baking tray in an even layer and coat with the remaining olive oil. Season with salt and black pepper and place in the oven. Bake for 10 minutes.

Take out the chicken of the refrigerator and thread it onto skewers. Place over the celery, pour in the chicken vegetable broth, and roast in the oven for 30 minutes.

Serve warm in plates.

NUTRITION: Cal: 579, Fat: 43g, Net Carbs: 6g, Protein: 39g

14 Spicy and Cheesy Turkey Dip

Ready in about 25 minutes | Servings 4

INGREDIENTS:

1 Fresno chili pepper, deveined and minced

1 ½ cups Ricotta cheese, creamed,

4% fat, softened

1/4 cup sour cream

1 tablespoon butter, room temperature

1 shallot, chopped

1 teaspoon garlic, pressed

1 pound ground turkey

1/2 cup goat cheese, shredded

Salt and black pepper, to taste

1 ½ cups Gruyère, shredded

DIRECTIONS:

Melt the butter in a frying pan over a moderately high flame.

Now, sauté the onion and garlic until they have softened. Stir in the ground turkey and continue to cook until it is no longer pink.

Transfer the sautéed mixture to a lightly greased baking dish. Add in Ricotta, sour cream, goat cheese, salt, pepper, and chili pepper.

Top with the shredded Gruyère cheese.

Bake in the preheated oven at 350 degrees F for about 20 minutes or until hot and bubbly in top.
Enjoy!

NUTRITION: 284 Calories; 19g Fat; 3.2g Carbs; 26.7g Protein; 1.6g Fiber

15 Spicy and Tangy Chicken Drumsticks

Ready in about 55 minutes | Servings 6

INGREDIENTS:

3 chicken drumsticks, cut into chunks

1/2 stick butter

2 eggs

1/4 cup hemp seeds, ground

 Salt and cayenne pepper, to taste

2 tablespoons coconut aminos

3 teaspoons red wine vinegar

2 tablespoons salsa

2 cloves garlic, minced

DIRECTIONS:

Rub the chicken with the butter, salt, and cayenne
pepper. Drizzle the chicken with the coconut aminos,
vinegar, salsa, and garlic. Allow it to stand for 30
minutes in your refrigerator. Whisk the eggs with the
hemp seeds. Dip each chicken strip in the egg
mixture. Place the chicken chunks in a parchment-
lined baking pan. Roast in the preheated oven at 390
degrees F for 25 minutes.

NUTRITION: 420 Calories; 28.2g Fat; 5g Carbs;
35.3g Protein; 0.8g Fiber

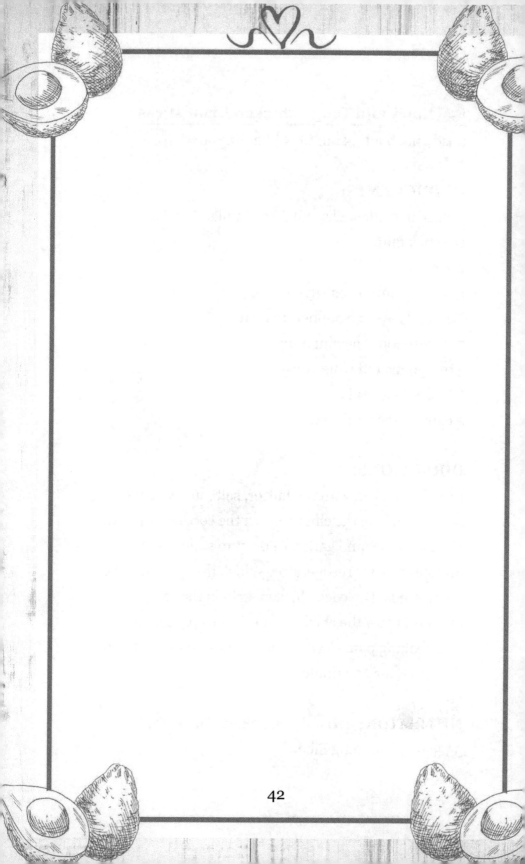

Beef Recipes

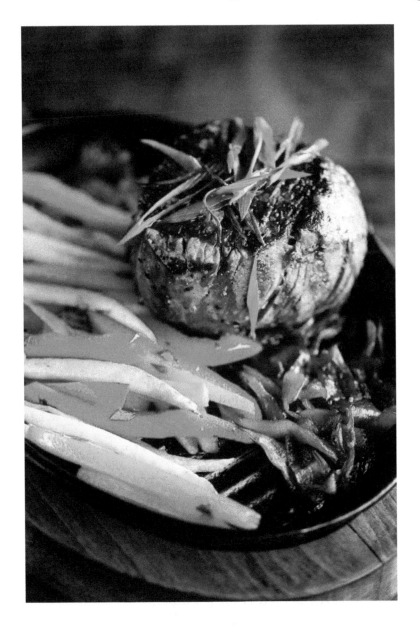

16 Parsley Steak Bites with Shirataki Fettucine

Total Time: approx. 30 minutes | 4 servings

INGREDIENTS:

2 (8 oz) packs shirataki fettuccine
1 lb thick-cut New York strip steaks, cut into 1-inch cubes
1 cup freshly grated Pecorino Romano cheese
4 tbsp butter
Salt and black pepper to taste
4 garlic cloves, minced
2 tbsp chopped fresh parsley

DIRECTIONS:

Boil 2 cups of water in a pot.
Strain the shirataki pasta and rinse well under hot running water.
Allow proper draining and pour into the boiling water.
Cook for 3 minutes and strain again.
Place a dry skillet and stir-fry the shirataki pasta until visibly dry, 1-2 minutes; set aside.
Melt butter in a skillet over medium heat, season the steaks with salt and pepper, and cook for 10 minutes.
Stir in garlic and cook for 1 minute.
Mix in parsley and shirataki; toss to coat.

Top with the Pecorino Romano cheese and serve.

NUTRITION: Cal 422; Net Carbs 7g; Fats 22g; Protein 36g

17 Classic Italian Bolognese Sauce

Ready in about: 35 minutes | Serves: 4

INGREDIENTS:

1 lb ground beef

2 garlic cloves, minced

1 onion, chopped

½ tsp dried oregano

½ tsp dried sage

½ tsp dried rosemary

14 oz canned diced tomatoes

2 tbsp olive oil

DIRECTIONS:

Heat olive oil in a saucepan. Add onion and garlic and cook for 3 minutes.

Add beef and cook until browned, about 4-5 minutes.

Stir in the herbs and tomatoes.

Cook for 15 minutes.

Serve with zoodles.

NUTRITION: Cal 318, Fat: 20g, Net Carbs: 5.9g, Protein: 26g

18   Beef Cheeseburger Casserole

Ready in about: 30 minutes | Serves: 6

INGREDIENTS:

3 tbsp olive oil
2 lb ground beef
1 cup cauli rice
2 cups cabbage, chopped
14 oz can diced tomatoes
1 cup Colby jack cheese, shredded

DIRECTIONS:

Preheat oven to 370°F.

Warm the olive oil in a pan over medium heat. Add in the ground beef and cook for 6 minutes until no longer pink.

Stir in the cauli rice, cabbage, tomatoes, and ¼ cup water.

Bring to boil and cook covered for 5 minutes until the sauce thickens.

Spoon the beef mixture into a baking dish and spread evenly.

Sprinkle with cheese and bake for 15 minutes until the cheese has melted. Remove and cool for 4 minutes.

Serve with zero carb crusted bread.

NUTRITION: Cal 385, Fat 25g, Net Carbs 5g, Protein 20g

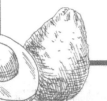
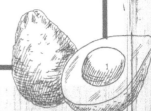

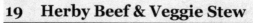

19 Herby Beef & Veggie Stew

Ready in about: 50 minutes | Serves: 4

INGREDIENTS:
1 lb stewed beef, cubed
2 tbsp olive oil
1 onion, chopped
2 garlic cloves, minced
14 oz canned diced tomatoes
¼ tsp dried oregano
¼ tsp dried basil
¼ tsp dried marjoram
Salt and black pepper to taste
2 carrots, sliced
2 celery stalks, chopped
1 cup vegetable broth

DIRECTIONS:
Warm the olive oil in a pan over medium heat. Add in the onion, celery, and garlic and sauté for 5 minutes. Place in the ground beef and stir-fry for 6 minutes. Mix in the tomatoes, carrots, vegetable broth, black pepper, oregano, marjoram, basil, and salt and simmer for 35 minutes.
Serve and enjoy!

NUTRITION: Cal 253, Fat 13g, Net Carbs 5.2g, Protein 30g

20   Beef with Grilled Vegetables

Ready in about: 30 minutes | Serves: 4

INGREDIENTS:

4 sirloin steaks

2 tbsp olive oil

3 tbsp balsamic vinegar

Vegetables

½ lb asparagus, trimmed

1 cup green beans

1 cup snow peas

1 red bell peppers, cut into strips

1 orange bell peppers, cut into strips

1 medium red onion, quartered

DIRECTIONS:

Set a grill pan over high heat. Grab 2 separate bowls
and put the beef in one and the vegetables in another.
Mix salt, pepper, olive oil, and balsamic vinegar in a
small bowl and pour half of the mixture over the beef
and the other half over the vegetables.

Coat the ingredients in both bowls with the sauce.
Place the steaks in the grill pan and sear both sides for
2-3 minutes each. When done, remove the beef onto a
plate; set aside.

Pour the vegetables and marinade in the pan and cook for 5 minutes, turning once. Share the vegetables into plates.

Top with beef, drizzle the sauce from the pan all over, and serve.

NUTRITION: Cal 515, Fat 32.1g, Net Carbs 5.6g, Protein 66g

Lamb Recipes

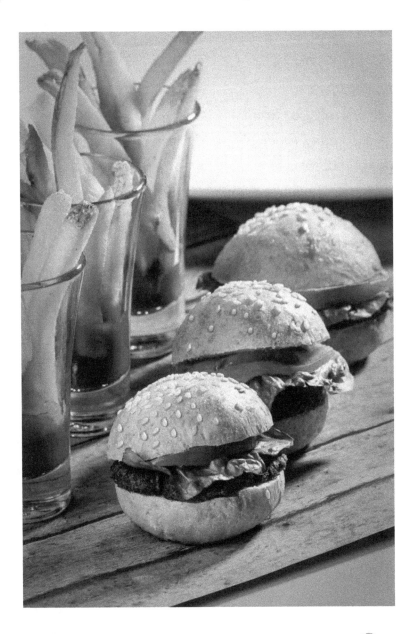

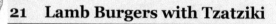

21   Lamb Burgers with Tzatziki

Prep time:20 min; Servings: 4

INGREDIENTS:

For burgers:

1 lb of grass-fed lamb

¼ cup chives finely chopped green onion or red onion if desired

1 Tbsp chopped fresh dill

½ tsp dried oregano or about 1 Tbsp freshly chopped

1 Tbsp finely chopped fresh mint

A pinch of chopped red pepper

Fine-grained sea salt

1 Tbsp water

tsp olive oil to grease the pan

For the tzatziki

*1 can of coconut milk with all the cooled fat and 1 Tbsp the discarded liquid portion ***

3 cloves of garlic

1 peeled cucumber without seeds, roughly sliced

Tbsp freshly squeezed lemon juice

2 Tbsp chopped fresh dill

3/4 tsp fine grain sea salt or to taste

Black pepper to taste.

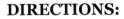

DIRECTIONS:

To make the tzatziki:

Put the garlic, cucumber, and lemon juice in food processor and press until finely chopped. Add the coconut cream, dill, salt, and pepper, and mix until well blended.

Put it in a jar with a lid and keep it in the refrigerator until it is served. The flavors become more intense over time when they cool in the fridge.

For burgers:

Thoroughly mix the ground lamb in a bowl with the chives or red onion, dill, oregano, mint, red pepper, and water.

Sprinkle the mixture with fine-grained sea salt and form 4 patties of the same size.

Heat a large cast-iron skillet over medium heat and brush with a small amount of olive oil. Lightly sprinkle the pan with fine-grain sea salt.

Place the patties into the pan and cook on each side for about 4 min, adjusting the heat to prevent the outside from becoming too brown. Alternatively, you can grill the burgers.

Remove from the pan and cover with tzatziki sauce.

NUTRITION: Cal 325 Fat: 15g, Net Carbs: 5g, Protein: 30g

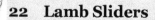

22 Lamb Sliders

Prep time:5 min; Servings: 6

INGREDIENTS:

1 lb minced lamb or half veal, half lamb

½ sliced onion

2 garlic cloves minced

1 Tbsp dried dill

1 tsp salt

½ tsp black pepper

DIRECTIONS:

Mix the ingredients gently in a large bowl until well combined. Overworking the meat will cause it to be tough.

Shape the meat into burgers.

Grill or fry in a pan over medium-high heat until cooked through, 4-5 min per side. If preparing in a pan, I like to quickly sear both sides then throw the burgers in a 350° F oven for 10 min to finish cooking through.

Serve with Tzatziki for dipping!

NUTRITION: Cal 216 Fat 17g Carbs 4.4g Protein 30G

23   Kofta

Prep time:15 min; Servings: 3-4

INGREDIENTS:

14 wooden skewers
2 Tbsp finely chopped garlic
¼ cup grated red onion
¼ cup chopped fresh parsley
¼ cup chopped fresh mint
1 Tbsp grated fresh ginger
½ tsp kosher salt
2 Tbsp Garam Masala
1 lb minced lamb
Greek flatbread
Chopped lettuce
Diced tomato
Tzatziki sauce

DIRECTIONS:

Put all the ingredients in a small container except the lamb until everything is combined. Then add the lamb and mix to combine without overloading the meat. Shape in seven oval patties.

Place 2 skewers next to each other (to facilitate the rotation of the grill).

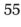

Roast over medium heat and change halfway to a well-sealed exterior and cook indoors to your liking. We prepared ours in the middle, which took about 12 to 15 min

To serve, place 1 or 2 patties on open flatbread and top with shredded lettuce, chopped tomato, and a generous drizzle of Tzatziki.

NUTRITION: Cal117 Fat: 5g, Net Carbs: 3g, Protein: 12g

24 Herb Koftas, Lamb and Red Onions

Prep time:15 min; Servings: 4

INGREDIENTS:

1 pound package lamb mince
1 red onion
2 garlic cloves, peeled
5 fresh mint leaves, washed and chopped
6-7 fresh petroleum leaves, washed and chopped
nice salt pinch
8 medium-sized wood skewers

DIRECTIONS:

Put the thin lamb in a bowl and season with the red onion and garlic. Add the chopped herbs and salt and blend to combine gently with your fingertips. Don't over-mix, or the meat may become tight and overworked.

Heat frying pan.

Take a skewer with 1 hand and take a small handful of the lamb mixture with the other side. Mold and pinch the meat around the rim, so it's a consistent thickness all the way.

Put in the heated pan gently. Continue with the mixture left. Add coconut or olive oil.

Turn the koftas regularly, brown on all sides, and cook for 10-12 min.

NUTRITION: Cal 259 Fat: 12.6g, Net Carbs: 4.4g, Protein: 31g

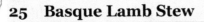

25   Basque Lamb Stew

Prep time:20 min; Servings: 4-6

INGREDIENTS:

3 ½ lbs shoulder of lamb, cut into 2-inch pieces

6 garlic cloves, crushed and peeled

1 sprig fresh rosemary, about 1 Tbsp minced meat

½ cup dry white wine

2 Tbsp extra virgin olive oil

1 large onion, peeled and chopped

leave

2 tsp sweet pepper

1 can 10 g roasted red peppers, cut into ½ inch strips

1 large ripe tomato, peeled, seeded and thinly sliced

2 Tbsp chopped fresh parsley

1 bay leaf

1 cup dry, full-bodied red wine

1 cup chicken broth

Freshly ground black pepper

DIRECTIONS:

Marinate the lamb with garlic, rosemary, and white wine: mix the lamb, half the garlic cloves, rosemary, and white wine in a medium bowl. Cook marinate for 2 to 3 hours.

Drain the meat, discard the marinade and dry with paper towels. Chop the remaining garlic cloves and store.

Brown the lamb: Heat the oil in a large, thick bottom pan with a lid, over medium heat. Work in batches, brown the meat everywhere, about 10 min per batch. Salt the meat while cooking.

Fry the onion and garlic: Remove the meat from the pan and add chopped onion to the pan. Boil, scrape the pieces of gold that are stuck to the bottom of the pot with a wooden spoon, until the onions are tender, about 5 min Add garlic and fry for another minute.

Return the meat to the pan, add pepper, roasted pepper, tomatoes, parsley, bay leaf, red wine, simmer: return the beef to pan with the onions and garlic. Add the bell pepper, roasted pepper, tomatoes, parsley, bay leaf, and red wine. Take to a boil, reduce the heat and simmer uncovered for 15 min, so that the liquids can slightly decrease.

Add chicken broth, simmer: Add chicken broth, boil, reduce heat and simmer, covered, occasionally stirring, until the meat is very soft, 2 to 2 ½ hours Add freshly ground black pepper and salt to taste.

NUTRITION: Cal 202 Fat: 9g, Net Carbs: 4g, Protein: 38g

Pork Recipes

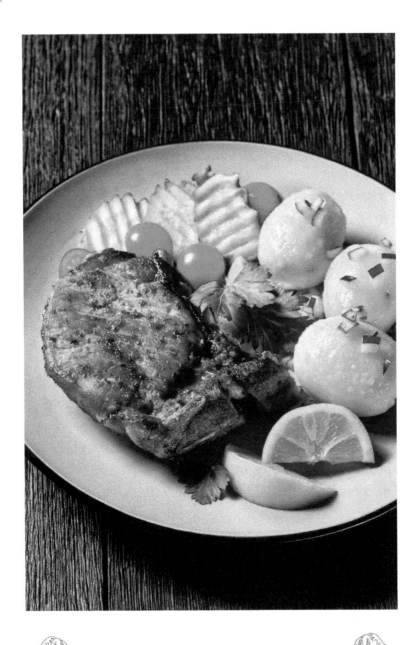

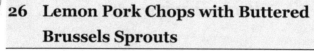

26 Lemon Pork Chops with Buttered Brussels Sprouts

Ready in about: 35 minutes | Serves: 6

INGREDIENTS:

3 tbsp lemon juice
3 cloves garlic, pureed
2 tbsp olive oil
6 pork loin chops
1 tbsp butter
1 lb Brussels sprouts, trimmed, halved
2 tbsp white wine
Salt and black pepper to taste

DIRECTIONS:

Preheat oven to 400°F. Mix the lemon juice, garlic, salt, black pepper, and oil in a bowl.

Brush the pork with the mixture. Place in a baking sheet and brown in the oven for 15 minutes, turning once. Remove.

Melt butter in a small wok and cook the Brussels sprouts for 5 minutes until tender.

Drizzle with white wine, sprinkle with salt and black pepper, and cook for another 5 minutes.

Serve them with the chops.

NUTRITION: Cal 549, Fat 48g, Net Carbs 2g, Protein 26g

27 Pulled Pork with Avocado

Ready in about: 2 hours 55 minutes | Serves: 6

INGREDIENTS

2 lb pork shoulder
1 tbsp avocado oil
½ cup vegetable stock
1 tsp taco seasoning
1 avocado, sliced

DIRECTIONS:

Preheat oven to 350°F. Rub the pork with taco seasoning and set in a greased baking dish.

Pour in the vegetable stock.

Place in the oven, cover with aluminum foil, and cook for 1 hour 45 minutes.

Discard the foil and cook for another 10-15 minutes until brown on top.

Leave to rest for 15-20 minutes. Shred it with 2 forks. Serve topped with avocado slices.

NUTRITION: Cal 567, Fat 42.6g, Net Carbs 4.1g, Protein 42g

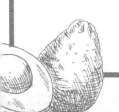
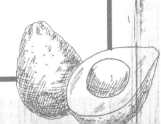

28   Smoked Pork Sausages with Mushrooms

Ready in about: 1 hour 10 minutes | Serves: 6

INGREDIENTS

3 yellow bell peppers, chopped

2 lb smoked sausage, sliced

Salt and black pepper to taste

2 lb portobello mushrooms, sliced

2 sweet onions, chopped

1 tbsp swerve sugar

2 tbsp olive oil

Arugula to garnish

DIRECTIONS:

Preheat oven to 320°F. In a baking dish, combine the sausages with swerve, olive oil, black pepper, onion, bell peppers, salt, and mushrooms. Pour in 1 cup of water and toss to ensure everything is coated. Bake for 1 hour. Remove and let sit for 5 minutes.
Serve scattered with arugula.

NUTRITION: Cal 525, Fat 32g, Net Carbs 7.3g, Protein 29g

29   Stuffed Pork with Red Cabbage Salad

Ready in about: 40 minutes + marinating time |
Serves: 4

INGREDIENTS

Zest and juice from 2 limes
2 garlic cloves, minced
¾ cup + 3 tbsp olive oil
1 cup fresh cilantro, chopped
1 tsp dried oregano
Salt and black pepper to taste
1 tsp cumin
4 pork loin steaks
2 pickles, chopped
4 ham slices
6 Swiss cheese slices
2 tbsp mustard
1 head red cabbage, shredded
2 tbsp vinegar
Salt to taste

DIRECTIONS:

In a food processor, blitz lime zest, ¾ cup oil,
oregano, cumin, cilantro, lime juice, garlic, salt, and
pepper. Rub the steaks with the mixture and toss to
coat. Place in the fridge for 2 hours. Arrange the

steaks on a working surface. Split the pickles, mustard, cheese, and ham on them, roll, and secure with toothpicks.

Heat a pan over medium heat. Add in the pork rolls, cook each side for 2 minutes and remove to a baking sheet. Bake in the oven at 350°F for 25 minutes. In a bowl, mix the cabbage with the remaining olive oil, vinegar, and salt. Serve with the meat.

NUTRITION: Cal 413, Fat 37g, Net Carbs 3g, Protein 26g

30 Paprika Pork Chops

Ready in about: 25 minutes | Serves: 4

INGREDIENTS

4 pork chops
Salt and black pepper to taste
3 tbsp paprika
¾ cup cumin powder
1 tsp chili powder

DIRECTIONS:

In a bowl, combine the paprika with black pepper, cumin, salt, and chili. Place in the pork chops and toss to coat.
Heat a grill to medium heat. Add in the pork chops and cook for 5 minutes.
Flip and cook for 5 minutes.
Serve with steamed vegetables.

NUTRITION: Cal 349, Fat 18.5g, Net Carbs 4g, Protein 41.8g

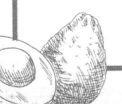

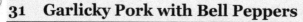

31   Garlicky Pork with Bell Peppers

Ready in about: 40 minutes | Serves: 4

INGREDIENTS

1 tbsp butter
4 pork steaks, bone-in
1 cup chicken stock
Salt and black pepper to taste
½ tsp lemon pepper
2 tbsp olive oil
6 garlic cloves, minced
4 bell peppers, sliced
1 lemon, sliced

DIRECTIONS:

Heat a pan with the olive oil and butter over medium heat.
Add in the pork steaks, season with black pepper and salt, and cook until browned; remove to a plate. In the same pan, add garlic and bell peppers.
Cook for 4 minutes.
Pour in the chicken stock, lemon slices, salt, lemon pepper, and pepper and stir for 5 minutes.
Return the pork steaks and cook for 10 minutes.
Pour the sauce over the steaks and serve.

NUTRITION: Cal 456, Fat 25g, Net Carbs 6g, Protein 40g

Fish and Seafood Recipes

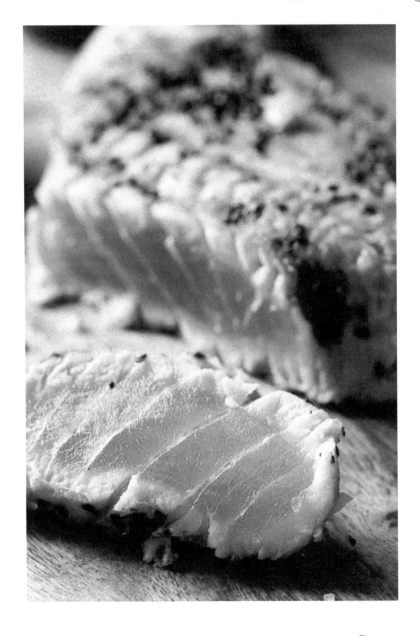

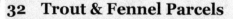

32   Trout & Fennel Parcels

Ready in about: 20 minutes | Serves: 4

INGREDIENTS:

1 lb deboned trout, butterflied
Salt and black pepper to taste
3 tbsp olive oil + extra for tossing
4 sprigs thyme
4 butter cubes
1 fennel bulb, thinly sliced
1 medium red onion, sliced
8 lemon slices
3 tsp capers

DIRECTIONS:

Preheat oven to 400°F. Cut out parchment paper wide
enough for each trout. In a bowl, toss the fennel and
onion with a little bit of olive oil and share into the
middle parts of the papers.

Place the fish on each veggie mound, top with a
drizzle of olive oil each, salt, pepper, 1 sprig of thyme,
and 1 cube of butter.

Lay the lemon slices on the fish. Wrap and close the
packets securely and place them on a baking sheet.
Bake in the oven for 15 minutes.

Garnish the fish with capers and serve.

NUTRITION: Cal 234, Fat 9.3g, Net Carbs 2.8g,
Protein 17g

33 Tuna Steaks with Shirataki Noodles

Ready in about: 30 minutes | Serves: 4

INGREDIENTS:

1 pack (7 oz) miracle noodle angel hair

3 cups water

1 red bell pepper, seeded and halved

4 tuna steaks

Salt and black pepper to taste

2 tbsp olive oil

2 tbsp pickled ginger

2 tbsp chopped cilantro

DIRECTIONS:

In a colander, rinse the shirataki noodles with running cold water.

Bring a pot of salted water to a boil. Blanch the noodles for 2 minutes. Drain and transfer to a dry skillet over medium heat.

Dry roast for a minute until opaque.

Grease a grill's grate with cooking spray and preheat to medium heat.

Season the red bell pepper and tuna with salt and pepper, brush with olive oil, and grill covered for 3 minutes on each side.

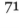

Transfer to a plate to cool. Assemble the noodles, tuna, and bell pepper into a serving platter.
Top with pickled ginger and garnish with cilantro.
Serve with roasted sesame sauce.

NUTRITION: Cal 310, Fat 18.2g, Net Carbs 2g, Protein 22g

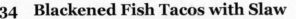

34   Blackened Fish Tacos with Slaw

Ready in about: 20 minutes | Serves: 4

INGREDIENTS:
1 tbsp olive oil
1 tsp chili powder
2 tilapia fillets
1 tsp paprika
4 low carb tortillas
Slaw
½ cup red cabbage, shredded
1 tbsp lemon juice
1 tsp apple cider vinegar
1 tbsp olive oil
Salt and black pepper to taste

DIRECTIONS:
Season the tilapia with chili powder and paprika. Heat the olive oil in a skillet over medium heat.
Add tilapia and cook until blackened, about 3 minutes per side. Cut into strips.
Divide the tilapia between the tortillas.
Combine all slaw ingredients in a bowl and top the fish to serve.

NUTRITION: Cal 523, Fat: 25g, Net Carbs: 3g, Protein: 35g

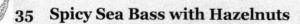

35   Spicy Sea Bass with Hazelnuts

Ready in about: 20 minutes | Serves: 2

INGREDIENTS:

2 sea bass fillets

2 tbsp butter, melted

⅓ cup roasted hazelnuts

A pinch of cayenne pepper

DIRECTIONS:

Preheat oven to 425°F. Line a baking dish with waxed paper.

Brush the butter over the fish. Process the cayenne pepper and hazelnuts in a food processor to achieve a smooth consistency.

Coat the sea bass with the hazelnut mixture. Place in the oven and bake for about 15 minutes.

Serve with mashed parsnips.

NUTRITION: Cal 467, Fat: 31g, Net Carbs: 2.8g, Protein: 40g

36 Parsley & Garlic Scallops

Total Time: approx. 30 minutes |6 servings

INGREDIENTS:

½ cup ghee, divided

2 lb large sea scallops

Salt and black pepper to taste

¼ tsp paprika

1 garlic clove, minced

3 tbsp water

1 lemon, zested and juiced

2 tbsp chopped parsley

DIRECTIONS:

Melt half of the ghee in a skillet, season the scallops with salt, pepper, paprika, and add to the skillet. Stir in garlic and cook for 4 minutes on both sides.

Remove to a bowl. Put remaining ghee in the skillet; add lemon zest, juice, and water.

Add in the scallops and cook for 2 minutes on low heat.

Serve the scallops sprinkled with parsley.

NUTRITION: Cal 258; Net Carbs 2g; Fat 22g; Protein 13g

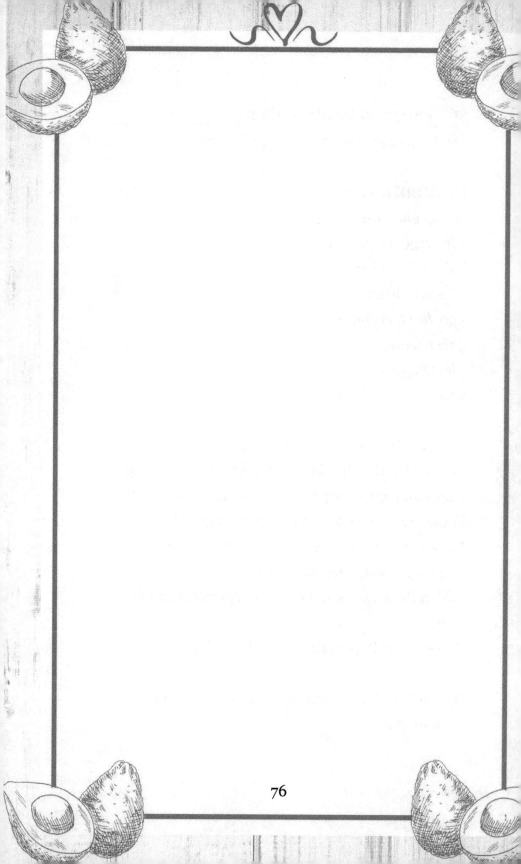

Vegetable Recipes

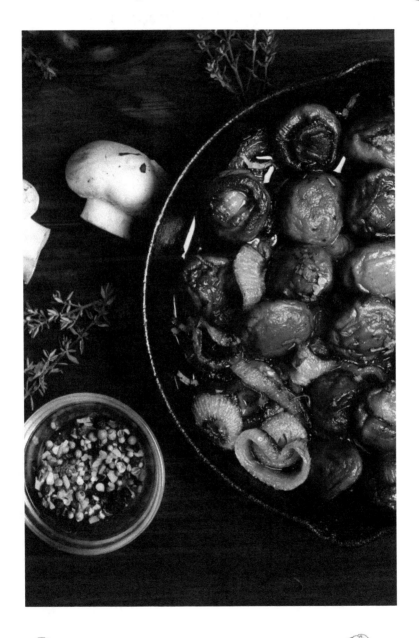

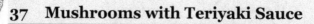

37   Mushrooms with Teriyaki Sauce

Prep time: 45 minutes | Cook time: 5 minutes
Serves 4

INGREDIENTS:

1½ pounds button mushrooms
¼ cup coconut milk
¼ cup dry wine
2 tablespoons sesame oil
1 tablespoon coconut aminos
1 teaspoon ginger-garlic paste
1 teaspoon red pepper flakes
Sea salt and ground black pepper, to taste
2 tablespoons roughly chopped fresh chives

DIRECTIONS:

In a bowl, stir together the mushrooms, coconut milk, wine, sesame oil, coconut aminos and ginger-garlic paste. Cover in plastic and let marinate in the refrigerator for 40 minutes.

Place the mushrooms along with the marinade in the Instant Pot. Season with the red pepper flakes, salt and black pepper.

Lock the lid. Select the Manual mode and set the cooking time for 5 minutes on High Pressure. When the timer goes off, perform a quick pressure release. Carefully open the lid.

Serve topped with the fresh chives.

NUTRITION: calories: 139 | fat: 11.1g | protein: 6.3g | carbs: 7.6g | net carbs: 5.2g

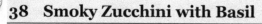

38 Smoky Zucchini with Basil

Prep time: 5 minutes Cook time: 4 minutes Serves 4

INGREDIENTS:

1½ tablespoons olive oil

2 garlic cloves, minced

1½ pounds (680 g) zucchinis, sliced

½ cup vegetable broth

1 teaspoon dried basil

½ teaspoon smoked paprika

½ teaspoon dried rosemary

Salt and pepper, to taste

DIRECTIONS:

Set the Instant Pot to the Sauté mode and heat the olive oil. Add the garlic to the pot and sauté for 1 minute, or until fragrant. Stir in the remaining ingredients.

Lock the lid. Select the Manual mode and set the cooking time for 3 minutes on Low Pressure. When the timer goes off, perform a quick pressure release. Carefully open the lid.

Serve immediately.

NUTRITION: calories: 81 | fat: 5.7g | protein: 2.3g | carbs: 6.9g | net carbs: 4.8g

39   Celery Croquettes with Chive Mayo

Prep time: 15 minutes | Cook time: 6 minutes | Serves 4

INGREDIENTS:

2 medium-sized celery stalks, trimmed and grated
½ cup of leek, finely chopped
1 tablespoon garlic paste
¼ teaspoon freshly cracked black pepper
1 teaspoon fine sea salt
1 tablespoon fresh dill, finely chopped
1 egg, lightly whisked
¼ cup almond flour
½ cup Parmesan cheese, freshly grated
¼ teaspoon baking powder
2 tablespoons fresh chives, chopped
4 tablespoons mayonnaise

DIRECTIONS:

Place the celery on a paper towel and squeeze them to remove excess liquid.

Combine the vegetables with the other ingredients, except the chives and mayo. Shape the balls using 1 tablespoon of the vegetable mixture.

Then, gently flatten each ball with your palm or a wide spatula. Spritz the croquettes with a non - stick cooking oil.

Air-fry the vegetable croquettes in a single layer for 6 minutes at 360°F (182°C).

Meanwhile, mix fresh chives and mayonnaise. Serve warm croquettes with chive mayo. Bon appétit!

NUTRITION: calories: 214 | fat: 18g | protein: 7g | carbs: 6.8g | net carbs: 5.2g

40   Cheddar Mushrooms with Wine

Prep time: 10 minutes | Cook time: 5 minutes | Serves 4

INGREDIENTS:

1 tablespoon olive oil

2 cloves garlic, minced

1 (1-inch) ginger root, grated

16 ounces Chanterelle mushrooms, brushed clean and sliced

½ cup unsweetened tomato purée

½ cup water

2 tablespoons dry white wine

1 teaspoon dried basil

½ teaspoon dried thyme

½ teaspoon dried dill weed

⅓ teaspoon freshly ground black pepper

Kosher salt, to taste

1 cup shredded Cheddar cheese

DIRECTIONS:

Press the Sauté button on the Instant Pot and heat the olive oil. Add the garlic and grated ginger to the pot and sauté for 1 minute, or until fragrant. Stir in the remaining ingredients, except for the cheese.

Lock the lid. Select the Manual mode and set the cooking time for 5 minutes on Low Pressure. When the timer goes off, perform a quick pressure release. Carefully open the lid..

Serve topped with the shredded cheese.

NUTRITION:

calories: 206 | fat: 13.7g | protein: 9.3g | carbs: 12.3g | net carbs: 7.1g | fiber: 5.2g

41　Green Cabbage in Cream Sauce

Prep time: 10 minutes | Cook time: 13 minutes |
Serves 4

INGREDIENTS:

1 tablespoon unsalted butter

½ cup diced pancetta

¼ cup diced yellow onion

1 cup chicken vegetable broth

1 pound (454 g) green cabbage, finely chopped

1 bay leaf

⅓ cup heavy cream

1 tablespoon dried parsley

1 teaspoon fine grind sea salt

¼ teaspoon ground nutmeg

¼ teaspoon ground black pepper

DIRECTIONS:

Press the Sauté button on the Instant Pot and melt the
butter. Add the pancetta and onion to the pot and
sauté for about 4 minutes, or until the onion is tender
and begins to brown.

Pour in the chicken vegetable broth. Using a wooden
spoon, stir and loosen any browned bits from the
bottom of the pot. Stir in the cabbage and bay leaf.

Lock the lid. Select the Manual mode and set the cooking time for 4 minutes on High Pressure. When the timer goes off, perform a quick pressure release. Carefully open the lid.

Select Sauté mode and bring the ingredients to a boil. Stir in the remaining ingredients and simmer for 5 additional minutes.

Remove and discard the bay leaf. Spoon into serving bowls. Serve warm.

NUTRITION:

calories: 211 | fat: 17.1g | protein: 7.2g | carbs: 7.3g | net carbs: 5.0g | fiber: 2.3g

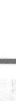
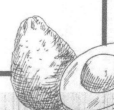

Soup Recipes

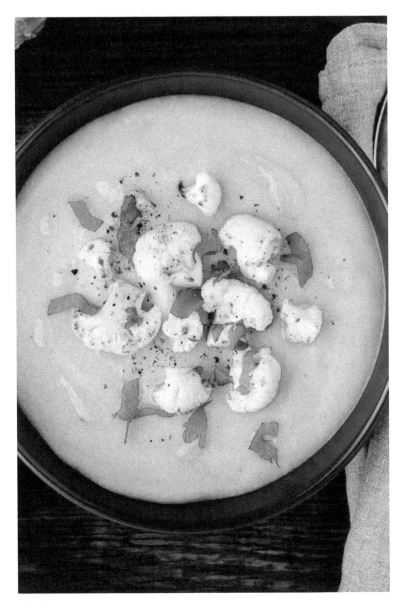

42   Creamy Cauliflower Soup with Bacon Chips

Ready in about: 25 minutes | Serves: 4

INGREDIENTS :

2 tbsp ghee

1 onion, chopped

2 head cauliflower, cut into florets

2 cups water

Salt and black pepper to taste

3 cups almond milk

1 cup white cheddar cheese, grated

3 bacon strips

DIRECTIONS:

Melt the ghee in a saucepan over medium heat and sauté the onion for 3 minutes until fragrant. Include the cauli florets and sauté for 3 minutes until slightly softened. Add the water and season with salt and black pepper. Bring to a boil and then reduce the heat. Cover and simme for 10 minutes.

Puree the soup with an immersion blender until the ingredients are evenly combined. Stir in the almond milk and cheese until the cheese melts. In a non-stick skillet over high heat, fry the bacon for 5 minutes until crispy. Divide soup between serving bowls, top with crispy bacon, and serve hot.

NUTRITION: Cal 402, Fat 37g, Net Carbs 6g, Protein 8g

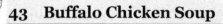

43   Buffalo Chicken Soup

Ready in about: 40 minutes | Serves: 4

INGREDIENTS:

2 chicken legs

2 tbsp butter, melted

1 onion, chopped

2 garlic cloves, minced

1 carrot, chopped

1 bay leaf

2 tbsp fresh cilantro, chopped

⅓ cup buffalo sauce

Salt and black pepper to taste

DIRECTIONS:

Add the chicken in a pot over medium heat and cover with water. Add in salt, pepper, and bay leaf. Boil for 15 minutes. Remove to a plate and let it cool slightly. Strain and reserve the broth.

Melt the butter in a large saucepan over medium heat. Sauté the onion, garlic, and carrot for 5 minutes until tender, stirring occasionally. Remove skin and bones from chicken and discard.

Chop the chicken and add it to the saucepan. Stir in the buffalo sauce for 1 minute and pour in the broth.

Bring to a boil. Cook for 15 minutes. Adjust the taste with salt and pepper and top with cilantro. Serve.

NUTRITION: Cal 215, Fat: 11.3g, Net Carbs: 2.4g, Protein: 7.5g

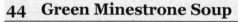

44   Green Minestrone Soup

Ready in about: 25 minutes | Serves: 4

INGREDIENTS:

2 tbsp ghee
2 tbsp onion-garlic puree
2 heads broccoli, cut into florets
2 celery stalks, chopped
4 cups vegetable broth
1 cup baby spinach
Salt and black pepper to taste
2 tbsp Gruyere cheese, grated

DIRECTIONS:

Melt the ghee in a saucepan over medium heat and sauté the onion-garlic puree for 3 minutes until softened. Mix in the broccoli and celery, and cook for 4 minutes until slightly tender.

Pour in the broth, bring to a boil, then reduce the heat to medium-low and simmer covered for about 5 minutes. Drop in the spinach to wilt, adjust the seasonings, and cook for 4 minutes. Ladle soup into serving bowls. Serve with a sprinkle of grated Gruyere cheese.

NUTRITION: Cal 227, Fat 20.3g, Net Carbs 2g, Protein 8g

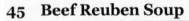

45 Beef Reuben Soup

Ready in about: 20 minutes | Serves: 6

INGREDIENTS:

1 onion, diced
6 cups beef stock
1 tsp caraway seeds
2 celery stalks, diced
2 garlic cloves, minced
2 cups heavy cream
1 cup sauerkraut, shredded
1 lb corned beef, chopped
3 tbsp butter
1 ½ cup swiss cheese, shredded
Salt and black pepper to taste

DIRECTIONS:

Melt the butter in a large pot. Add onion, garlic, and celery and fry for 3 minutes until tender. Pour the beef stock over and stir in sauerkraut, salt, caraway seeds, and add a pinch of black pepper.

Bring to a boil. Reduce the heat to low, and add the corned beef. Cook for about 15 minutes, adjust the seasoning. Stir in heavy cream and cheese and cook for 1 minute.

NUTRITION: Cal 450, Fat: 37g, Net Carbs: 8g, Protein: 23g

46 Slow Cooker Beer Soup with Cheddar & Sausage

Ready in about: 8 hr | Serves: 6

INGREDIENTS:

1 cup heavy cream

10 oz sausages, sliced

1 celery stalk, chopped

1 carrot, chopped

2 garlic cloves, minced

4 oz cream cheese, softened

1 tsp red pepper flakes

6 oz low carb beer

2 cups beef stock

1 onion, chopped

1 cup cheddar cheese, grated

Salt and black pepper to taste

DIRECTIONS:

Turn on the slow cooker. Add in beef stock, beer, sausages, carrot, onion, garlic, celery, salt, red pepper flakes, and pepper and stir well. Pour in enough water to cover all the ingredients by roughly 2 inches. Close the lid and cook for 6 hours on Low. Open the lid and stir in the heavy cream, cheddar, and cream cheese and cook for 2 more hours. Ladle the soup into bowls and serve. Yummy!

NUTRITION: Cal 244, Fat: 17g, Net Carbs: 4g, Protein: 5g

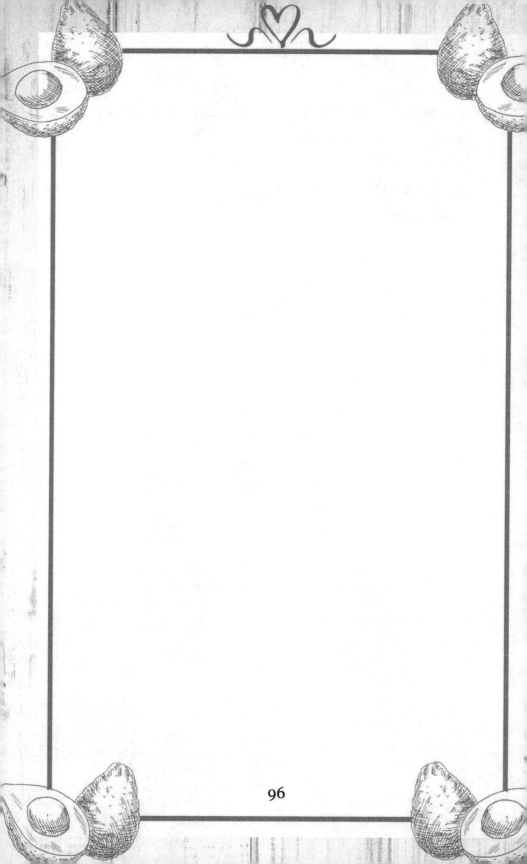

Dessert Recipes

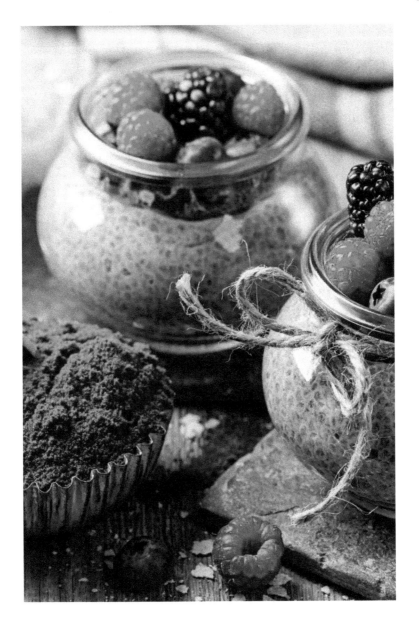

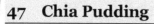

47 Chia Pudding

Total Time: approx. 20 min + cooling time|4 servings

INGREDIENTS:

4 tbsp chia seeds

½ cup almond milk

1 cup coconut cream

½ cup sour cream

½ tsp vanilla extract

¼ tsp cardamon powder

1 tbsp stevia

DIRECTIONS:

Add all the ingredients in a mixing bowl and stir to combine. Leave to rest for 20 minutes. Apportion the mixture among bowls. Serve and enjoy!

NUTRITION: Cal 258; Net Carbs: 2g; Fat: 24g; Protein: 5g

48   Peanut Dark Chocolate Barks

Total Time: approx. 10 min + cooling time|6 servings

INGREDIENTS:

10 oz unsweetened dark chocolate, chopped

¼ cup toasted peanuts, chopped

¼ cup dried cranberries, chopped

½ cup erythritol

DIRECTIONS:

Line a baking sheet with parchment paper. Pour
chocolate and erythritol in a bowl, and microwave for
25 seconds. Stir in cranberries, peanuts, and salt,
reserving a few cranberries and peanuts for
garnishing. Pour the mixture on the baking sheet and
spread out. Sprinkle with remaining cranberries and
peanuts. Refrigerate for 2 hours to set. Break into
bite-size pieces to serve.

NUTRITION: Cal 225; Net Carbs 3g; Fat 21g;
Protein 6g

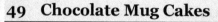

49 Chocolate Mug Cakes

Total Time: approx. 5 minutes | 2 servings

INGREDIENTS:

2 tbsp ghee

1 ½ tbsp cocoa powder

2 tbsp erythritol

1 egg

2 tbsp almond flour

1 tbsp psyllium husk powder

2 tsp coconut flour

½ tsp baking powder

A pinch of salt

DIRECTIONS:

In a bowl, whisk the ghee, cocoa powder, and erythritol until a thick mixture forms. Whisk in the egg until smooth and then add in almond flour, psyllium husk, coconut flour, baking powder, and salt. Pour the mixture into 2 medium mugs and microwave for 70 to 90 seconds or until set.

NUTRITION: Cal 92; Net Carbs 1.8g; Fat 12g; Protein 8.2g

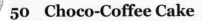

50   Choco-Coffee Cake

Total Time: approx. 30 minutes|4 servings

INGREDIENTS:

3 tbsp golden flaxseed meal, ground

1 tbsp melted butter

1 cup almond flour

2 tbsp coconut flour

1 tsp baking powder

¼ cup cocoa powder

¼ tsp salt

½ tsp espresso powder

1/3-½ cup coconut sugar

¼ tsp xanthan gum

¼ cup organic coconut oil

2 tbsp heavy cream

2 eggs

DIRECTIONS:

Preheat oven to 400 F. Grease a springform pan with melted butter. In a bowl, mix almond flour, flaxseed meal, coconut flour, baking powder, cocoa powder, salt, espresso, coconut sugar, and xanthan gum. In another bowl, whisk coconut oil, heavy cream, and eggs. Combine both mixtures until smooth batter forms. Pour the batter into the pan and bake until a toothpick comes out clean, 20 minutes.

Transfer to a wire rack, let cool, slice, and serve.

NUTRITION: Cal 232; Net Carbs 6.3g; Fat 22g; Protein 5.5g

51   Chocolate Bark with Almonds

Ready in about: 5 minutes + cooling time | Serves: 12

INGREDIENTS:

½ cup toasted almonds, chopped

½ cup butter

10 drops stevia

¼ tsp salt

½ cup unsweetened coconut flakes

4 oz dark chocolate

DIRECTIONS:

Melt together the butter and chocolate, in the microwave, for 90 seconds.

Remove and stir in stevia. Line a cookie sheet with waxed paper and spread the chocolate evenly.

Scatter the almonds on top, coconut flakes, and sprinkle with salt.

Refrigerate for one hour.

NUTRITION: Cal 161, Fat: 15.3g, Net Carbs: 1.9g, Protein: 1.9g

CPSIA information can be obtained
at www.ICGtesting.com
Printed in the USA
BVHW051019070921
616210BV00002B/298

9 781956 289114